TABLE OF *Contents*

DISCLAIMER

The materials and content contained in this book are not intended to be a substitute for professional medical advice, diagnosis, or treatment. All recommendations in this book should be presented to your health care provider prior to implementing them. The writer of this book makes no warranties or representations, express or implied, as to the accuracy or completeness, timeliness or usefulness of any opinions, advice, services or other information contained or referenced in this book. Additionally, the writer of this book does not assume any risk for your use of this book, or any information contained therein. The writer reserves the right to update or change information contained in this book at any time. In consideration of your use of this book, you agree not to take risks beyond your level of experience, aptitude, training, and comfort level. You also agree that in no event will the writer or any other party involved in creating or delivering this book or any site linked to this book, be liable to you in any manner whatsoever for any decision made or action or non-action taken by you in reliance upon the information provided. Any action you take upon the information on this book is strictly at your own risk and the writer is not liable for any losses and damages in connection with the use of this book. While the writer strives to provide only quality information and links to helpful and ethical websites, we have no control over the content and nature of these sites and the links to other websites do not imply a recommendation for all the content found on these sites. Disclosure: You should assume that the writer of this book is an affiliate for providers of goods and services mentioned in this book. The owner may be compensated when you purchase after clicking on a link.

INTRODUCTION

Hey Quarantine Cuties!

As much as I have enjoyed the extra family time and decreased social obligations, I didn't enjoy the part where I had begun to feel less healthy mentally, physically, and spirituality. For many of us, this current situation has increased our "scroll time", decreased our physical activity, and made us a little less happy and a lot more fearful. Especially during times like these, investing in your health becomes extremely important. As an avid gym-goer, this time made it imperative for me to readjust my workout routine. This is how Quarantine Curves (QC) was born. QC was initially designed to act as my workout guide. But now, I'm divulging those secrets to you. A lot of these are my personal, favorite go-to exercises, so let's stay healthy together.

QC is a glute-focused workout plan that can be followed at home, due to the readily available and accessible equipment that is used. The objective of QC is to provide a simple, easy-to-follow guide to help and empower you. I hope that this book will facilitate the start of your own incredible health journey so that eventually you can modify and create your path.

I hope you enjoy it as much as I do and thank you for your support!

GLUTE *Institute*

Having a better understanding of why you do what you do, makes you empowered. I would feel like I failed you, if I didn't clarify some things in this book before we move to the workout phase.

WHAT CAN YOU TELL ME ABOUT THE GLUTES?

When you think glutes, you may think of just one body part. Although the gluteus maximus is mainly responsible for the general shape of our derriere, it's only one portion that makes up what some call their glutes. Our glutes are actually made up of three muscles: the gluteus maximus, gluteus medius, and gluteus minimus. The medius is located above the maximus, and the minimus is located below. So when I use the term "glutes", I'm referring to the gluteus maximus and the two smaller muscles that make up our derrière.

GLUTE *Institute*

CAN WORKING OUT MY GLUTES MAKE THEM BIGGER/LOOK BETTER?

Several individuals who look to regularly exercise their glutes and achieve significant growth primarily do so for aesthetic purposes. In simpler words, many people exercise their glutes to get a nice and curvy bum, so it is very possible to accentuate your glutes through exercise. While the rate of progress and maximum growth potential is determined partly by your natural genetics, it is possible to significantly change the shape of your buttocks through exercise. These aesthetic improvements occur when you make changes to your cross-sectional glute muscle area, leading to a rounder, perkier, and more athletic appearance. That's not all! Exercising your glute muscles can also improve the overall state of your body by building muscle and decreasingfat.

ARE THERE ANY PRACTICAL REASONS TO EXERCISE MY GLUTES?

While an attractive aesthetic is the main motivator behind glute training, some people target these particular muscles for health and recovery reasons. For example, glute training can have a positive impact on a person's knees, keeping them in a strong and stable position when running, jumping, and landing. Unstable knee joints can collapse inwards and cause serious injuries, including anterior cruciate ligament tears. Strong glute muscles can also promote positive hip extension. Moreover, they also relieve the stress on your back when lifting heavy weights, something that could otherwise lead to serious backpain.

GLUTE *Institute*

WHAT ABOUT MY UPPER BODY?

Many people make the mistake of assuming that glute exercises only work the lower body around your derriere. However, the majority of these workouts help in training parts of your upper body and core too. Therefore, even if you follow this training plan, which only includes glute- based exercises, you will still come out of it with some upper- body/corestimulus. Having said that, it is always a good idea to pair this up with a few specific exercises directed towards these areas.

GLUTE *Institute*

IS THERE ONE SPECIFIC EXERCISE THAT IS IDEAL FOR GLUTE GROWTH? WHAT IS THE SECRET?

Hip thrusts and squats are two of the most effective tools to use on the path towards improved glutes. However, one of the **best** ways to train your glutes and achieve consistent growth is via the hip thrust. Studies have demonstrated that this exercise **alone** results in a significant increase in glute growth and improvements. Hip thrusts are found to be more effective than squats in growth and bodily improvements in certain instances.

SO CAN I DO HIP THUSTS ONLY ?

Yes, you can! Hip thrusts are awesome. However, when done alone, they will not provide the most well-rounded glutes and you would miss out on several other benefits mentioned earlier that accompany a well-rounded glute training program. This is why we offer different options with our workouts.

GLUTE *Institute*

ANY FINAL THOUGHTS ON THE BENEFITS OF A WELL-ROUNDED GLUTE PROGRAM?

I mentioned squats and hip thrusts earlier, and both of them target the prime movers and trunk stabilizers, as well as a number of other key muscle groups within the body. Prime movers include the glutes, adductor magnus, and the majority of your hamstring muscles, while the trunk stabilizers include the erector spinae and other muscles in your core. However, I haven't even mentioned the amazing benefits of deadlifts, extensions, and abduction exercises which are also included in this book. So, take the time to see all of the wonderful exercises QC has to offer!

Book Specific F.A.QS

ARE YOU SOME KIND OF GLUTE EXPERT?

Haha no, not at all. I'm a nurse, so naturally, I focus on overall health. However, I am very interested in glute building. For years, I've researched information on glute development due to my personal interest. QC is just a mini-compilation of that knowledge and experience. I'm hands-on and visual, so I just wanted something quick and easy to follow during this interesting period, and decided to share what I have developed, with you.

WHAT APPROACH DOES QC USE?

QC utilizes a lower weight, higher rep approach. Since most of us do not have access to commercial equipment during these trying times (including myself), it was determined that this is the best approach.

HOW CAN I GET MY GLUTES BIGGER WITHOUT BIG WEIGHTS?

When I started working out, even I believed that low reps and big lifts were the only way to gain muscle. However, thanks to evidence-based research, I discovered that it is not the only way. For example, researchers at Mcalester University conducted a study comparing the strength and muscle gain of two different groups. One group lifted light weights for up to 25 reps, and the other group lifted heavier weights for up to 12 reps. The study concluded that the lighter weights were just as effective in building muscle, and that both groups were comparable in strength.

WHAT ARE GLUTE ACTIVATIONS?

Before each exercise, there are 2 glute activation exercises. The purpose of these exercises is to warm-up and not to wear out your muscles. These exercises prepare your glutes for the more intensive workouts later.

WHAT ARE BURNOUTS?

Burnouts are optional exercises performed at the end of a workout to fatigue your muscles. Burnouts promote hypertrophy and transport blood to the glutes. This can be a little advanced for some people, so you need not start with them immediately, or even practice them during every session.

HOW MANY DAYS A WEEK SHOULD I WORKOUT?

The program is set up in such a way that you work out on alternate days every week, amounting to 4 days in total. However, if you want to want to work out only 2 or 3 days a week, you can choose to do so, provided, you are not cheating yourself. Also, variety can be a good thing. So you don't necessarily have to push yourself 100% to fatigue every day and you shouldn't.

STRETCH

Stretching can be beneficial when performed before and after a workout. Stretching can help improve flexibility, increase range of motion, and increase blood flow to muscles, in addition to providing several other health benefits. There are 2 types of stretching we will consider; dynamic and static stretching.

DYNAMIC STRETCHING

Dynamic stretches are warm-ups that prepare your muscles for future performance, which sometimes include performing certain movements. Oftentimes, these exercises could mimic your workout but at a lower intensity. So, this could include gentle arm swings, walking lunges, or a light jog.

STATIC STRETCHING

Static stretching is a form of stretching that should be performed following physical activity, but it's contraindicated prior to your workout. Static stretching occurs when a position is maintained for about 45 seconds. Think yoga poses.

NUTRITION

Nutrition plays a huge role in determining your results. I'd have to write a separate book to explain nutrition in a detailed manner. However, I've included some vital information for you to keep in mind.

According to Health.gov, females aged 14 and up need anywhere from 1,800-2,200 calories/day, and males need 2,200-2,800 calories/day, depending on age and activity level.

Age	Sedentary	Mod. Active	Active
13	1,600	2,000	2,000
14-18	1,800	2,000	2,400
19-20	1,200	2,200	2,400
21-25	1,200	2,200	2,400
26-30	1,800	2,000	2,400
31-40	1,800	2,000	2,200
36-50	1,800	2,000	2,200
51	1,600	1,800	2,200

BREAKING DOWN YOUR GOALS:

In order to **lose weight**, you would need to consume fewer calories than what you use. "Eating just 150 calories more a day than you burn can lead to an extra 5 pounds over 6 months. That's a gain of 10 pounds a year." (National Institute of Mental Health, 2013)

In order to **gain weight**, you need to consume more calories than what you use, since eating extra calories results in a build-up of stored body fat and weight gain.

Nutrition **Cont.**

A healthy eating plan provides your body with the nutrients required to function normally while balancing calories and lowering the risk of diseases. In other words, eating healthier can contribute to increased energy, better skin, and overall better health.

If you want to take a big step toward your health, you may want to consider cutting out or limiting one or all of these:

> SUGARS

> ALCOHOL

> PROCESSED FOODS

> DAIRY

> BREAD

> HIGH SODIUM

> CARBONATED BEVERAGES

I know it's easier said than done, that's why I snuck in a few healthy snack ideas for you at the end of this book. lol

IMPORTANT *Tips*

> Rest for about 30 seconds between each set.

> Push through your heels.

> Remember to exhale on exertion. In other words, inhale while lowering, and exhale when rising/pushing etc.

> Begin with as many reps as you can safely perform without struggling beyond a certain safe limit. If it's too difficult, you can just do 2 sets, but push as much as you safely can and don't give up!

> Remember to SQUEEZE your glutes while performing these exercises.

IMPORTANT *Tips*

Really try to mentally focus on the muscles you are trying to target. Sometimes it helps to put your hand on the area that you are trying to target to see what area you're actually engaging.

PROGRESSIVE OVERLOAD

You will eventually begin to notice some results, but they won't be as effective if you do not incorporate **progressive overload.** This is just a fancy term for **making your muscles work harder with each workout.** You do this by **increasing reps and/or sets or increasing weight.**

Ways to increase weight: Ankle weights, resistance bands, water jugs, your baby etc.

You get the picture! Remember, you won't continue to gain if you remain stagnant with your workout routine. You won't gain by staying the same. That'll preach! lol

IMPORTANT *Tips*

KEEP A JOURNAL OF YOUR PROGRESS

> Record the number of reps and sets you do

> Record how you feel

> If you want to take it a step further, record your food intake

TAKE PICTURES BEFORE, DURING, AND AFTER

> Take pictures from the front, side, and back.

> Try to wear the same clothing for your progress pictures.

> Take pictures at the same time everyday, preferably before you eat in themorning.

GLUTE ACTIVATION

DAY 1&3 G&L DAY

Donkey Kicks 3 sets/10 reps

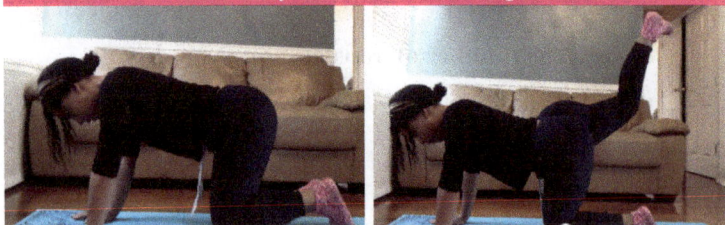

- Position yourself on all fours
- Kick your leg behind you with your knee bent
- Retrace your leg back to the starting position and repeat until reps are complete.
- Repeat numbers 1-4 with the opposite leg.

Fire Hydrants 3 sets/10 reps

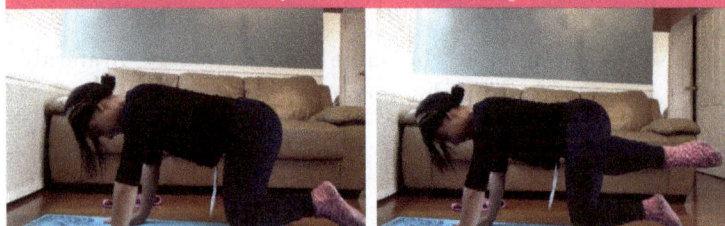

- Position yourself on all fours
- Extend your leg out to side with your knee remaining bent
- Lower your leg but do not touch the ground. Raise leg again and repeat the motion until reps are complete.

GLUTES & LEGS

DAY 1&3 G&L DAY

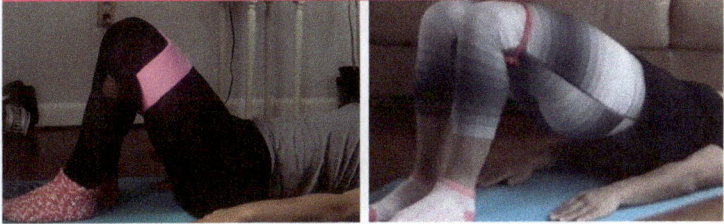

Banded Glute Bridge 3 sets/20-25 reps

- Lay on your back and fold your knees while your feet
- remain flat on the floor
- Separate your feet, making band tight.
- Lift your hips high up until your glutes no longer touch
  the ground. Squeeze glutes, and pause for a moment
- Slowly lower your hips back to the ground

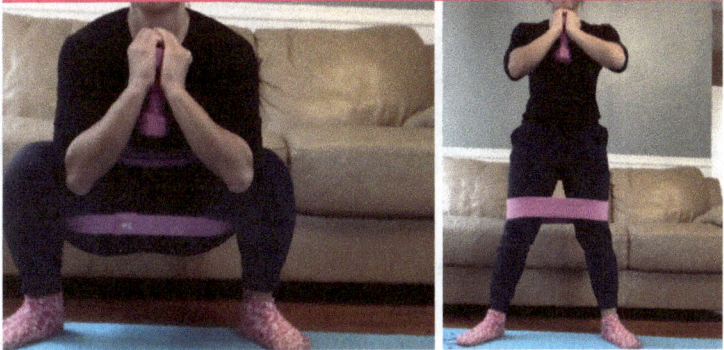

Goblet Squat 3 sets/20-25 reps

- Although I am using a band here, start without one initially
- Hold item in a manner mimicking the image
- Position yourself in a squat ensuring your chest stays up
  with elbows pushing out against the inside of your knees
- Return to the starting position

GLUTES & LEGS CONT.

DAY 1&3 G&L DAY

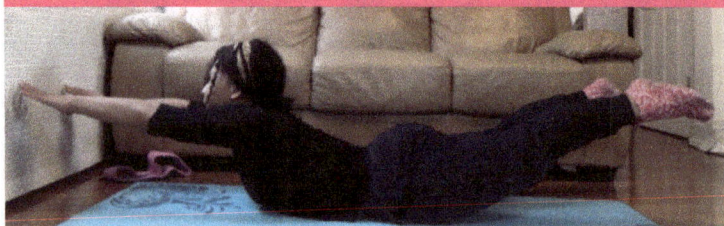

Superman 2 sets/20-25

- Lay on your stomach on the floor
- Lift legs using hamstrings and glute muscles, while simultaneously lifting your torso and stretching out your arms
- Hold for a moment and slowly return to the starting position

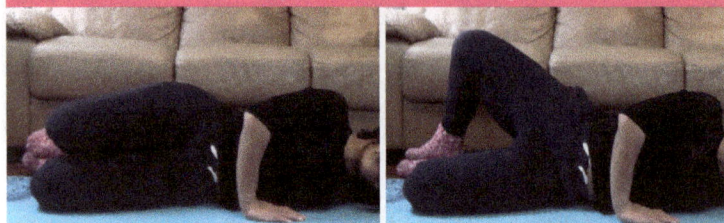

Fire Hydrants 3 sets/10 reps

- Lay on your side.
- Bend knees and bring them forward stacking your feet.
- Lift your top knee while your feet remain touched.
- Lower your top leg back down and repeat until reps are complete.

OPTIONAL BURNOUT

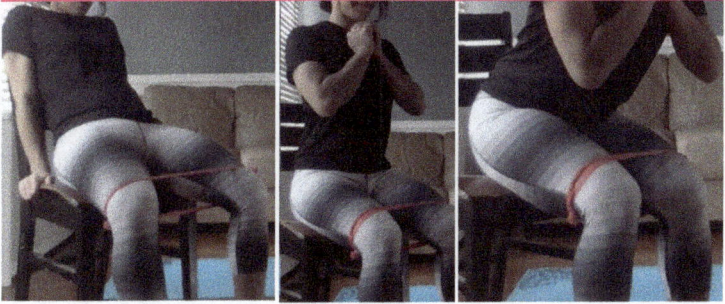

- In a seated position, place band above knees and separate feet to provide tension
- Lean back
- Separate knees and bring your knees back together until reps are completed
- Sit upright and begin the previous step immediately until reps are completed
- Lean forward and immediately do the third step for desired reps

Glute Bridge / Abduction 2-3 minute

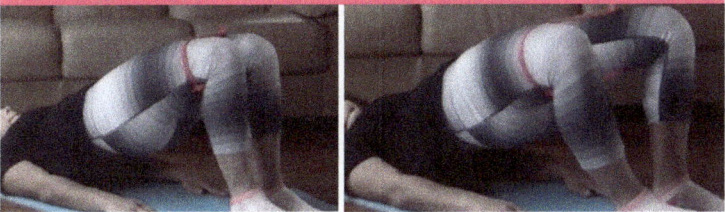

- With band placed above knees perform several glute bridges
- While hips are still raised or when hips are lowered back to the ground, separate knees for several reps
- You want to feel the exercise burning your muscles.
- Perform this exercise for 3 minutes

GLUTE ACTIVATION

DAY 2&4 G&L DAY

Side to side lunges 3 sets/10 reps each side

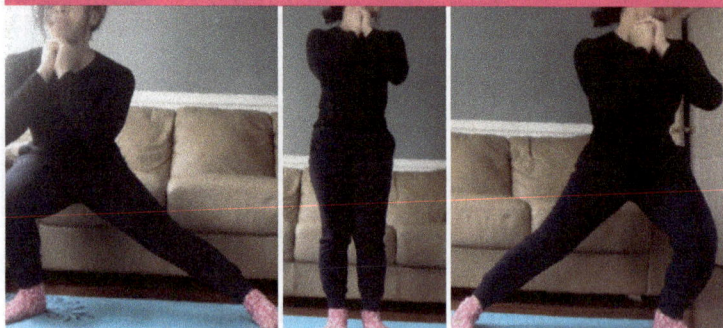

- Begin in a standing position
- Shift your weight to your right leg lowering your body and bending your right knee
- Shift your weight to your left side without fully returning to standing position
- Repeat this motion for desired reps.

Standing kickbacks 3 sets/10 reps

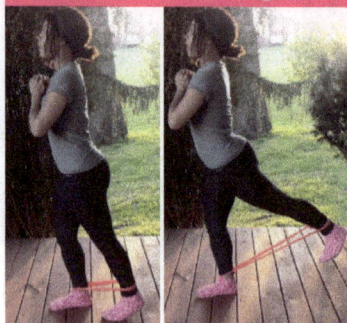

- With feet shoulder-width apart, kick your leg out behind you squeezing glutes.
- Slowly lower leg to original position.
- Repeat for desired reps
- Repeat on opposite leg.

GLUTES & LEGS

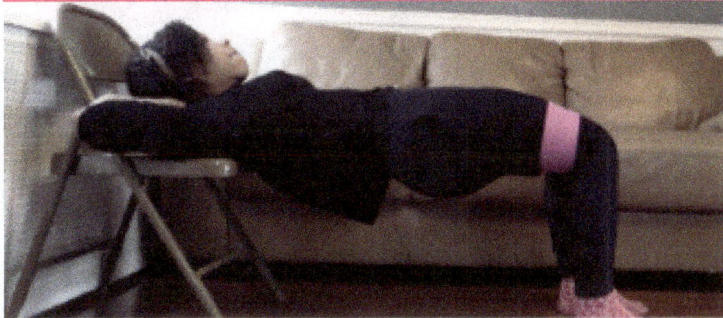

Hip Thrusts 3 sets/20-25 reps

- Though I used the chair for a better angle, the couch is better-suited for this routine
- Put your shoulders on a surface with arms straight out to the side and knees bent
- Raise hips and squeeze glutes tightly
- Open knees while turning feet on the edge
- Bring knees back together while squeezing
- Slowly lower to the bottom

Step-up 3 sets 10-12 reps each leg

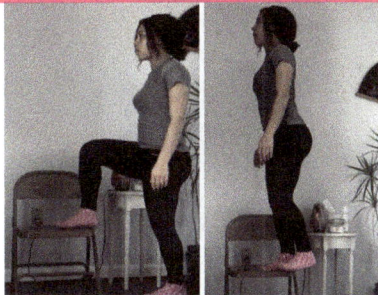

- Place your foot on a surface that is positioned at a higher level (close to your knees), while pressing your foot
- Allow the opposite foot to follow, so you are now standing on the surface
- Return to the starting position, beginning with the initiating foot and let your other foot follow, to stand on the floor
- Repeat with the starting leg until reps are complete
- Repeat motion on opposite leg

LEG DAY CONT.

DAY 2&4 LEG DAY

Reverse Hyper 3 sets 20-25 reps

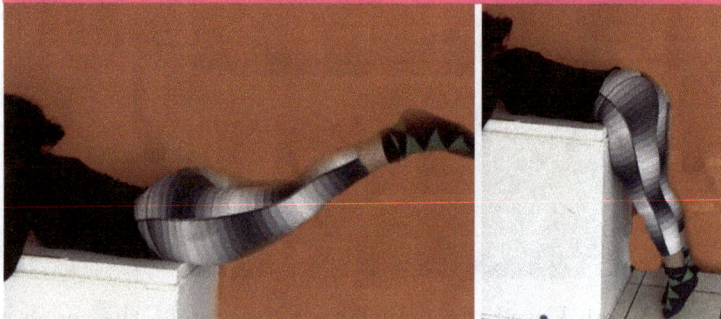

- Lay torso and waist on a raised platform with feet raised above the floor, while legs continue to remain straight
- Raise your legs up by extending your hips as high as possible until legs are nearly straight.
- Lower legs to original position.
- Repeat until reps are complete

Standing Hip Abduction 3 sets 20 -25 reps

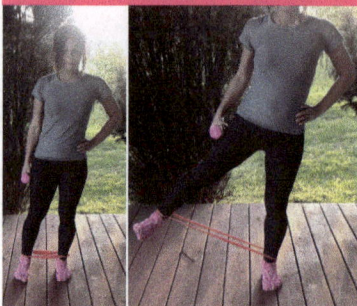

- Stand with your feet shoulder width apart.
- Raise one leg to the side
- Slowly return to starting position.
- Repeat until reps are complete
- Repeat on opposite leg

OPTIONAL BURNOUT

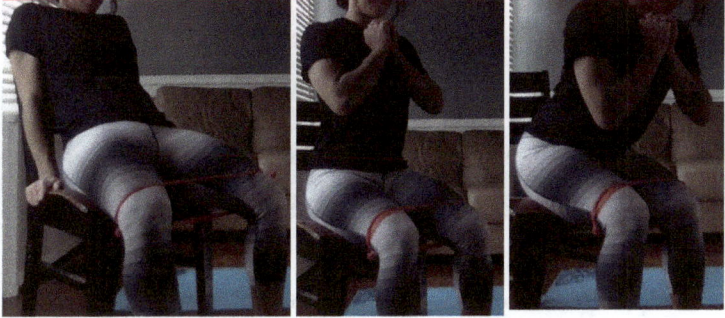

- In a seated position, place band above knees and separate feet to provide tension
- Lean back
- Separate knees and bring your knees back together until reps are completed
- Sit upright and begin the previous step immediately until reps are completed
- Lean forward and immediately do the third step for desired reps

Glute Bridge / Abduction 2-3 minute

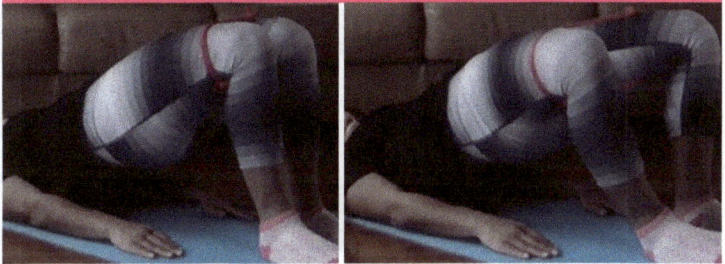

- With band placed above knees perform several glute bridges
- While hips are still raised or when hips are lowered back to the ground, separate knees for several reps
- You want to feel the exercise burning, perform this exercise for 3 minutes

GLUTE ACTIVATION

DAY 1&3 G&L DAY

Frog Glute Bridge 2 sets/10 reps

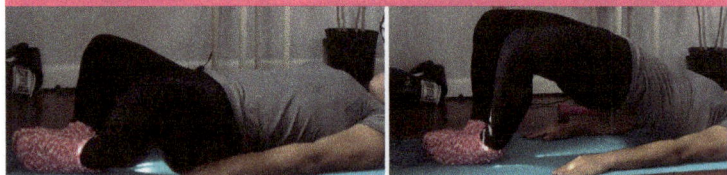

- Lay on your back
- Separate feet making band tight.
- Lift your hips high, squeeze glutes, and pause for a moment
- Slowly lower your hips back to the ground

Banded Side to Step Squats 2 sets/10 reps

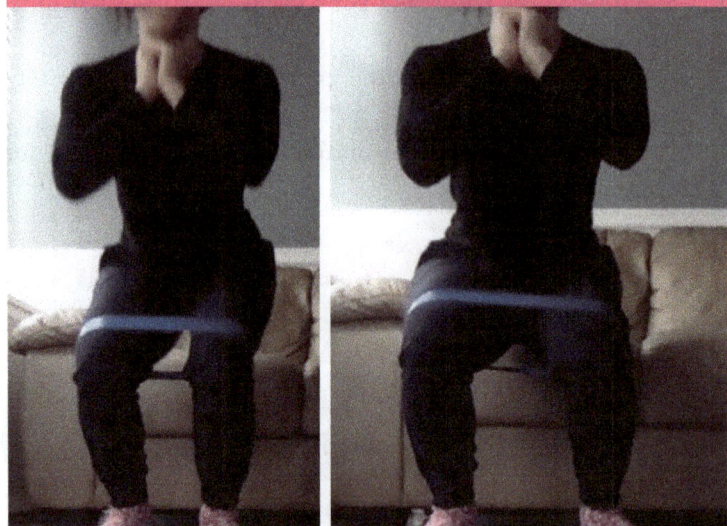

- With band above knees position yourself in a squat
- Step to one side and then return to starting position\Step to opposite side and return to starting position
- Repeat this motion for desired reps

GLUTES & LEGS

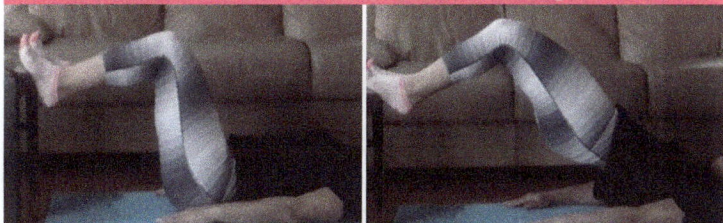

Elevated Glute Bridge 3 sets 20-25 eps

- Place feet on an elevated surface while lying on the floor
- Lift your hips up as high as possible
- Squeeze your glutes and slowly lower to starting position
- Repeat for desired reps

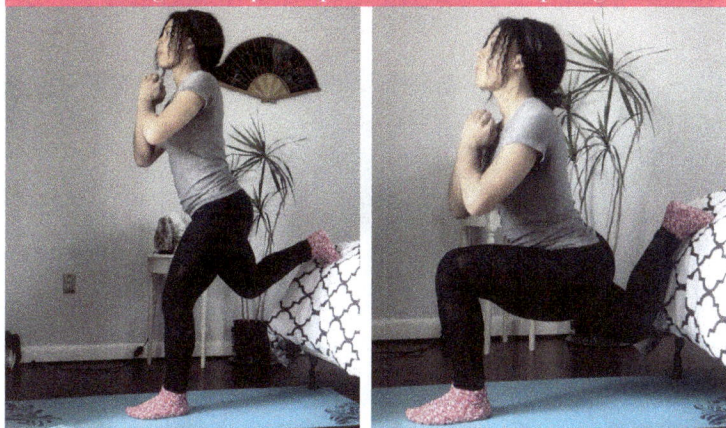

Bulgarian Split Squat 3 sets/10-12 reps leg

I would recommend a lower surface than what is depicted in the picture.

- Elevate one foot on a surface behind you
- Bend your front knee and lower your back knee towards the floor
- Push back up through the heel of your front foot to return to the starting position,
- Repeat on the opposite leg for desired reps on the other leg

GLUTES & LEGS CONT.

DAY 1&3 G&L DAY

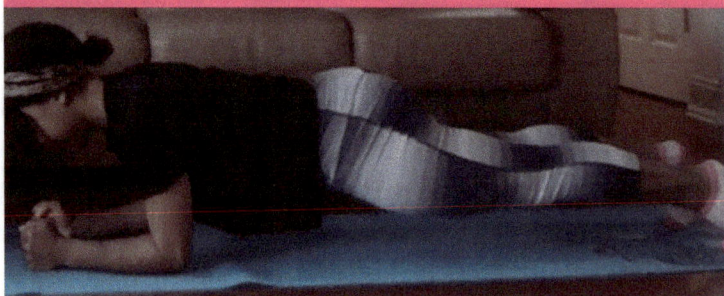

Plank 2 sets 15-30 sec

- With your forearms on the ground, back flat and lifted off the floor, and your toes on the floor, engage your core and squeeze your glutes.

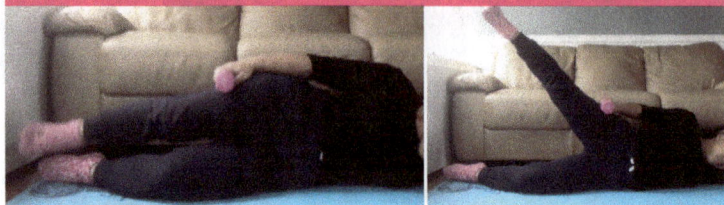

Lying Hip Abduction 3 sets/20-25 reps

- Lay on your side
- Lift your leg up
- Slowly lower back down
- Repeat for the desired reps
- Repeat on the opposite leg
- Continue the motion until desired reps are completed

OPTIONAL BURNOUT

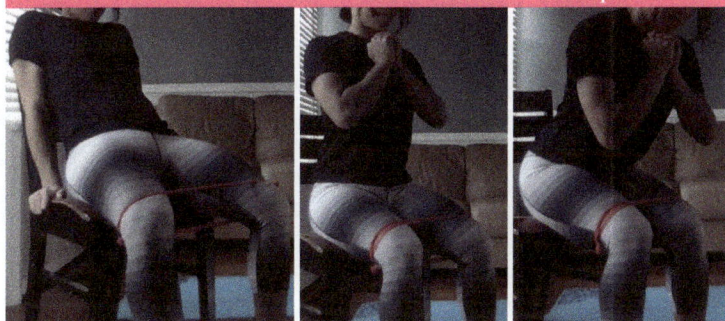

Tri Position Seated Abduction 3 sets/20 reps

- In a seated position, place band above knees and separate feet to cause tension
- Lean back
- Separate knees and bring your knees back together until reps are completed
- Sit upright and begin the previous step immediately until reps are completed
- Lean forward and immediately do the third step for desired reps

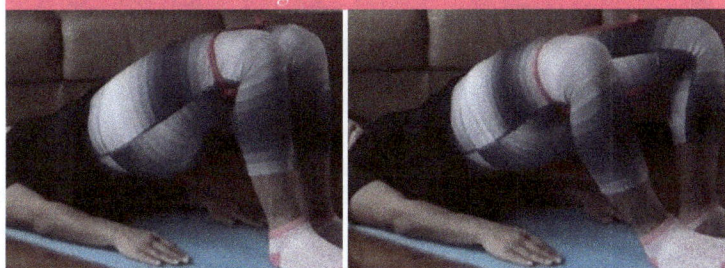

Glute Bridge / Abduction 2-3 minute

- With band placed above knees perform several glute bridges
- While hips are still raised or when hips are lowered back to the ground, separate knees for several reps
- You want to feel the exercise burning, perform this exercise for 3 minutes

GLUTE ACTIVATION

DAY 2&4 G&L DAY

Squat Jack 3 sets/10 reps

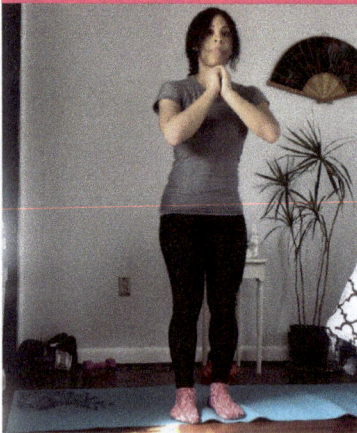

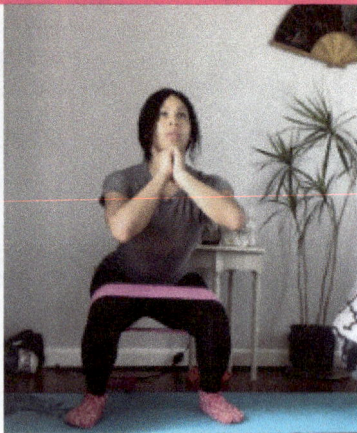

- Clasp hands together in front of your chest.
- Jump to extent your feet out, push your hips back, and bend your knees into a squat.
- Bring your feet back together while in a squat

Rainbow Kicks 3 sets/10 reps/leg

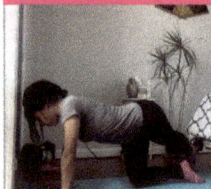

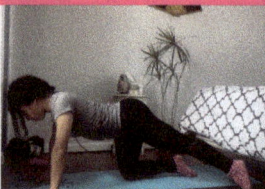

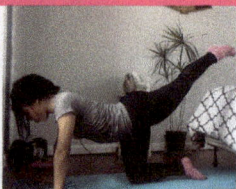

- While on all fours, extend one leg in an outward direction without bending your knee
- Lift your leg up as high as possible squeezing your glutes
- Without twisting your hips, bring your leg to opposite side
- Slowly return to the starting position and repeat for desired reps
- Repeat this motion for the opposite leg when you have completed all your reps

GLUTES & LEGS

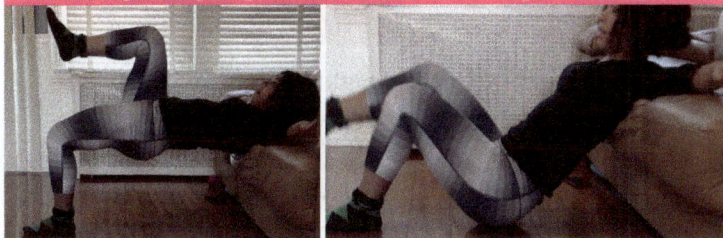
Single-Leg Hip Thrust 3 sets/10-12 reps each leg

- Place your back on a surface with one knee bent and your glutes positioned on the floor
- Raise the opposite leg to resemble a '7,'while raising your hips until they are in line with your torso
- Remember to really squeeze the glutes tightly
- Slowly lower back to the starting position and repeat until reps are complete
- Repeat with the opposite leg
- Continue the motion until desired reps are completed

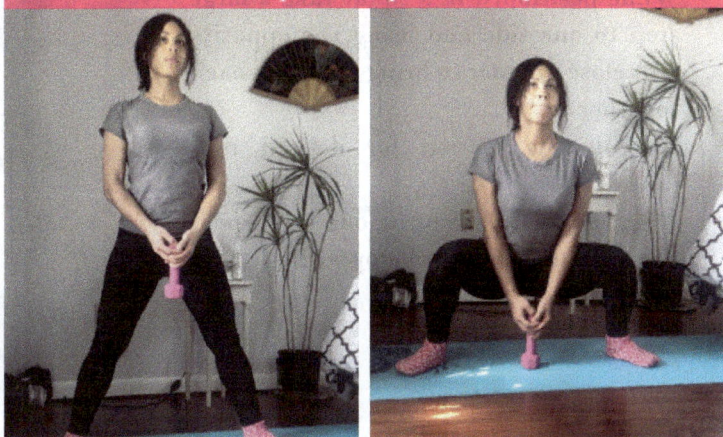
Sumo Squats 3 reps /20-25 reps

- Stand with feet wider than shoulder-width apart Perform a squat

GLUTES & LEGS

DAY 2&4 G&L DAY

Stiff-Legged RDL 3 X10-12 reps

- Hold a dumbbell or a weighted item in each hand, keeping your arms straight in front of your thighs
- With knees slightly bent, slowly bend at your hip joint making sure to keep your back straight
- Slowly lower the weights as far as you possibly can go without arching your back, while the item remains close to your legs
- Squeeze your glutes in order to pull yourself back up
- Repeat until reps are complete

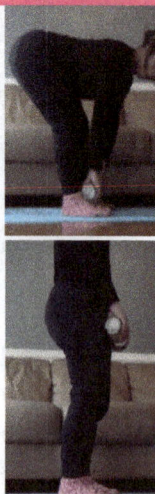

Banded Side to Step Squats 2 sets/10 reps

- While positioned in a squat take a large step to one side and bring the opposite foot close in order to bring your feet back together
- Repeat this motion for desired reps desired
- After completing reps on one leg, repeat the same motion on the opposite leg for desired reps

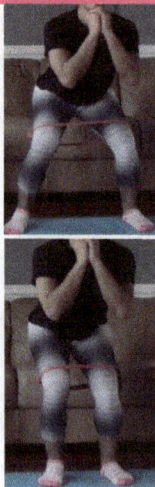

OPTIONAL BURNOUT

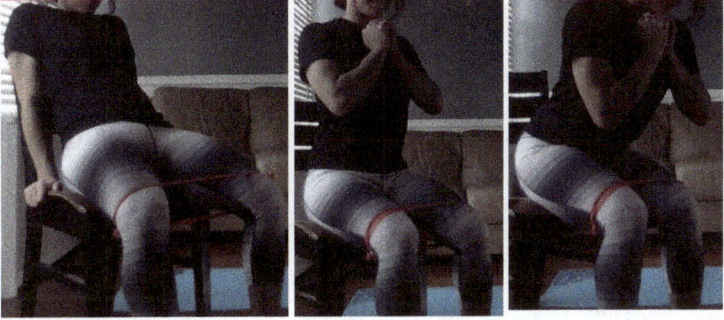

- In a seated position, place band above knees and separate feet to create tension
- Lean back
- Separate knees and bring your knees back together until reps are completed
- Sit upright and begin the previous step immediately until reps are completed
- Lean forward and immediately do the third step for desired reps

Glute Bridge / Abduction 2-3 minute

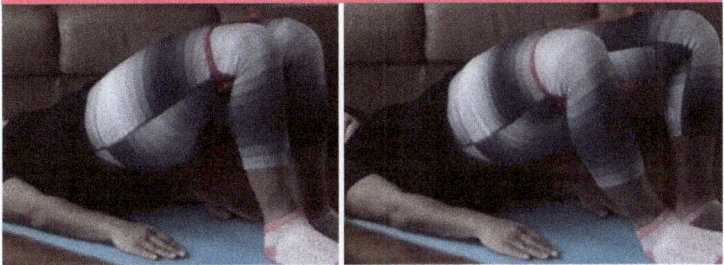

- With band placed above knees perform several glute bridges
- While hips are still raised or when hips are lowered back to the ground, separate knees for several reps
- You want to feel the exercise burning, perform this exercise for 3 minutes

NEED MORE *Inspiration?*

Once again, I want you to be empowered, so here are more options.

If you want to get creative with your own glute routine, it should be well-rounded, targeting different areas. In other words, you can do something like this.

1. Hip thrust-like workout
2. Squat-Like Workout
3. Deadlift/Extension Workout
4. Side Workout

This is just a basic template, which you can use to perform many different types of workouts as it can be easily modified.

1. If you're feeling lazy or are limited by time constraints, you can just try a hip-thrust-only workout like this.

2. Do 10 hip thrusts pausing at the top for 5 seconds before going back down

3. Immediately do 10 single leg hip-thrusts

4. Repeat step 1

Perform another 10 rep hip thrusts on the opposite leg from earlier.

I said this is a lazy workout, but you are still really going to feel this! This workout is definitely not as well-rounded, but if you need a quick exercise to show your glutes some love you can try to get results with this as well.

NEED MORE *Inspiration?*

Deadlift/Extension Alternatives

Single-Leg Hip Hinges with Dowel

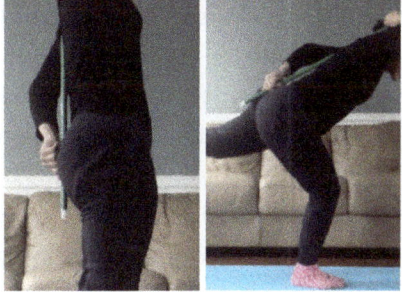

- Place an item similar to a broomstick againsts your back ensuring that contact is maintained with your head, mid-back, and tail bone, at all times
- Balance on one leg and hinge at the hip pushing your glutes back
- Lower your upper body as far as you can whilst maintaining those points of contact
- Using the muscles of the back of the leg, pull yourself up Squeeze your butt once you are upright

Single-Leg Bulgarian Hip Hinge

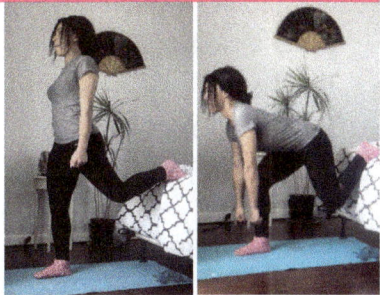

- With feet hip-width apart, place one foot on a surface behind you.
- With knees soft and a straight back push hips and hamstrings back as you hinge at the hips
- Squeeze your glutes to rise back up

- Anchored Pull Through Using Resistance Band
- With a straight back reach down to grab band
- Using glutes and hamstrings, squeeze to rise back up, pause and squeeze
- Hinge forward without curving back to repeat movement for desired reps without returning tothe

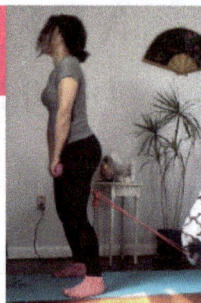

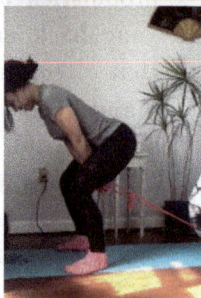

Kettlebell Swing Variation

- I just love this exercise because it's fun to me lol
- With feet shoulder-width apart and knees slightly bent hold a kettlebell or another weighted item (preferably using a two-handed, overhand grip)
- Bend your hips back until the item is between your legs
- Squeeze glutes to bring yourself back up
- Reverse the momentum
- Continue until reps are complete

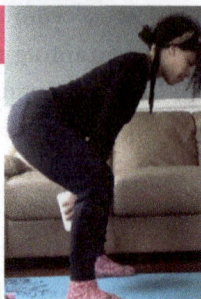

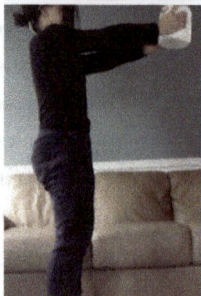

NEED MORE *Inspiration?*

Side Exercise Alternatives

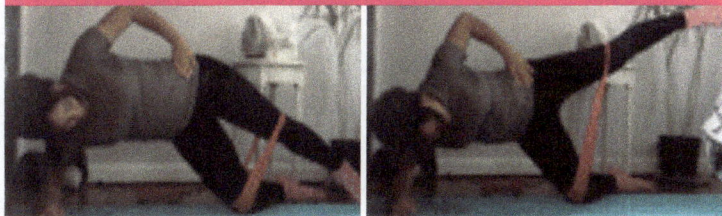

Side-Lying Raised Hip Abduction

Similar to the side-lying abduction. In this exercise, you can raise your hips to increase the difficulty level.

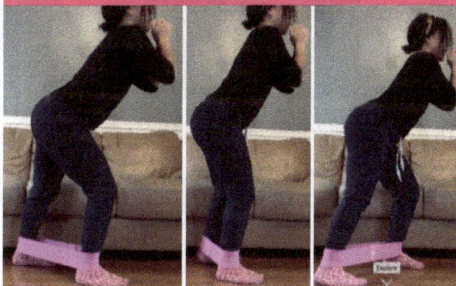

Angled Step Back

Instead of stepping straight back , you can step back to a 45--degree angle to give yourself a different kind of workout.

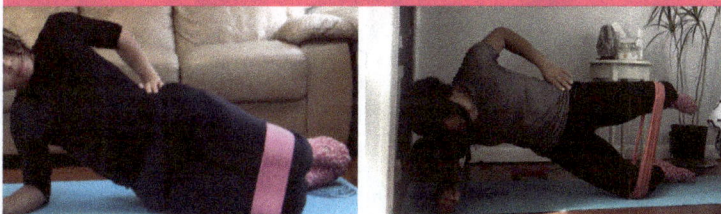

Elevated Clam

Similar to the clamshell. In this exercise, you can raise your hips to increase the difficulty level.

NEED MORE *Inspiration?*
More Random Exercises

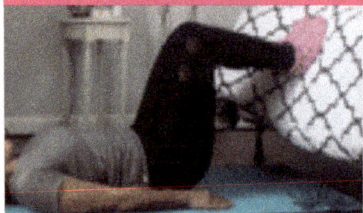
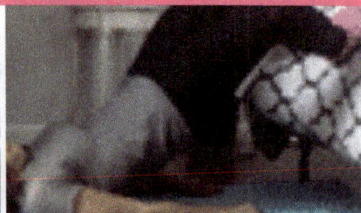

Elevated Frog Glute Bridge

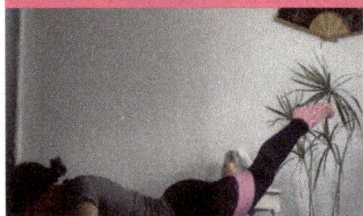
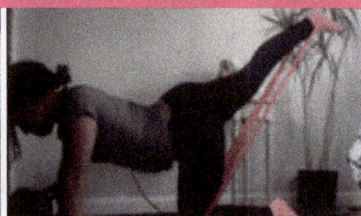

Banded Kickback Variations

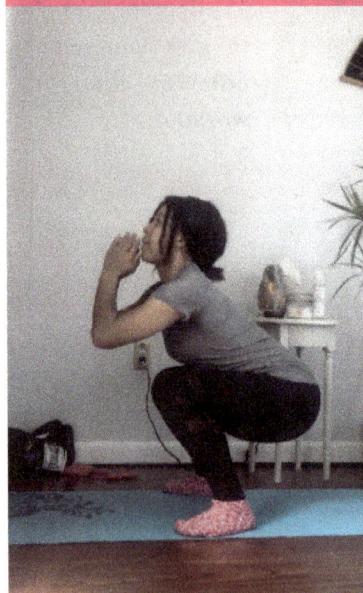
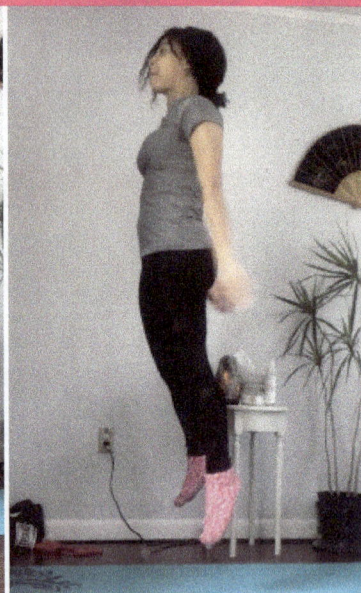

Jump Squats

Curtsy Lunge

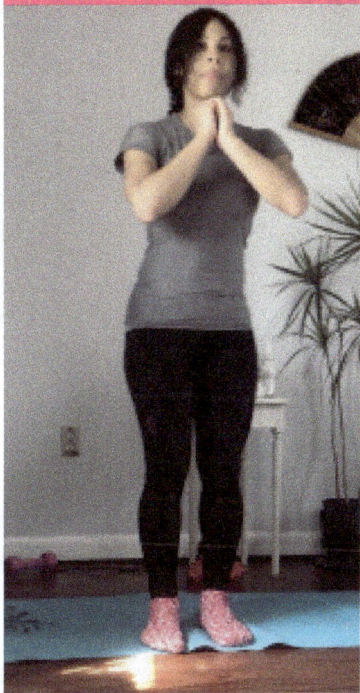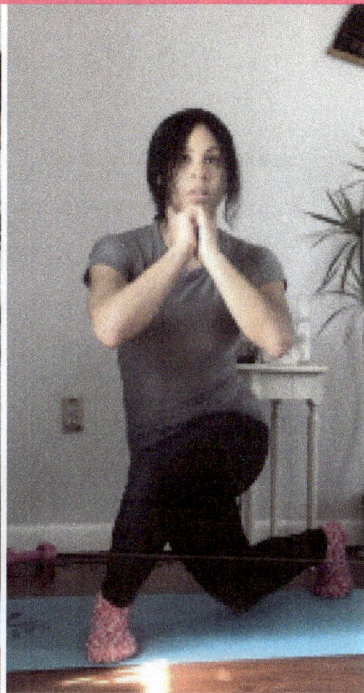

Calf-Raises

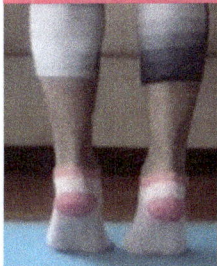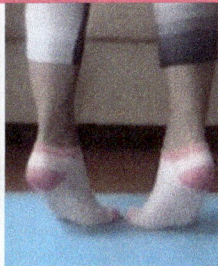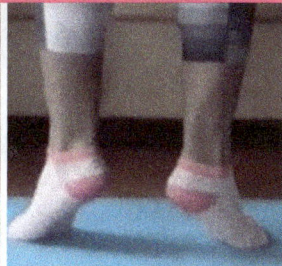

NEED MORE *Inspiration?*

As promised here are some snack ideas

> Peanut butter and celery

> Peanut butter and apples

> Watermelon

> Greek yogurt and berries

> Homemade Kale Chips

> Homemade Sweet Potato Fries

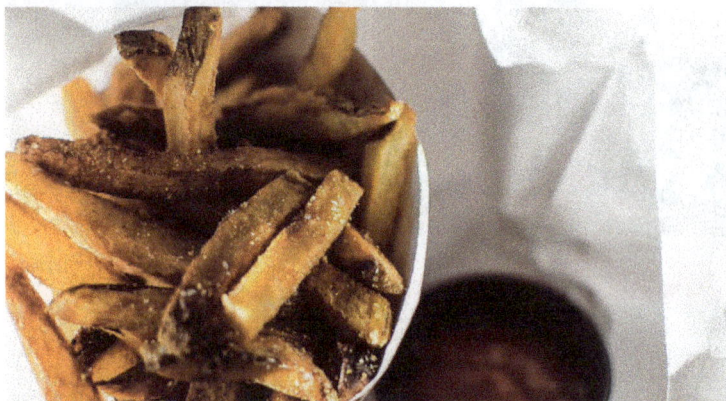

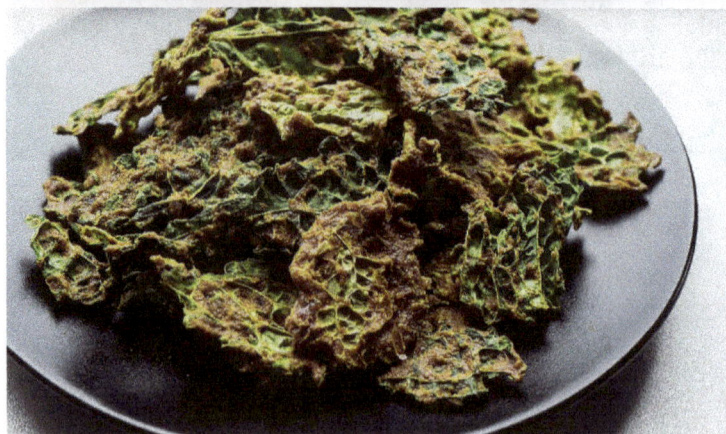

NEED MORE *Inspiration? Cont.*

KALE CHIPS

Ingredients

- 1 bunch kale
- 2 teaspoons olive oil
- 1 tablespoon nutritional yeast
- 1 tablespoon water
- 1/8 teaspoon salt
- A pinch of cayenne

Directions

Remove the kale stems and chop leaves, put to the side. Mix the rest of the ingredients and spread the mixture onto kale. You can set the oven to 200 and leave it baking for about 45 minutes, or if you want to keep a close eye on it, you can set it to 400 degrees and cook for 10 minutes

SWEET POTATO FRIES

Ingredients

- 3 sweet potatoes
- 1 teaspoon coconut oil
- Spices added for taste:
- Rosemary
- Black pepper
- Sea salt

Directions

Set oven to 300. Spread coconut oil on the baking sheet. Cut sweet potato into 1/8 of inch slices. Place slices on the baking sheet. Add spices. Bake until brown on both sides (about 30 mins)

Gasp. I know, I know! You're wondering where all the yummy fatty foods and meats are. Don't worry, you DO NOT have to give up on all meats and snacks in order to be healthier. *gasp* I know. Instead, you can incorporate a better way of eating. For example, the Mediterranean diet, which includes yummy food and meats, has been associated with better brain function, lower blood pressure, better cholesterol, more stable blood sugar among a whole host of other benefits. Here, you can take a quiz and get a personalized plan with real-time calculations and recipes to see if it is something you want to consider: https://bit.ly/2zNzDc4

REFERENCES

Abade, Eduardo, Nuno Silva, Ricardo Ferreira, Jorge Baptista, Bruno Gonçalves, Sofia Osório, and João Viana. "Effects of Adding Vertical or Horizontal Force-Vector Exercises to In-season General Strength Training on Jumping and Sprinting Performance of Youth Football Players." *Journal of Strength and Conditioning Research*, 2019, 1. doi:10.1519/jsc.0000000000003221.

"Appendix 2. Estimated Calorie Needs per Day, by Age, Sex, and Physical Activity Level." Appendix 2. Estimated Calorie Needs per Day, by Age, Sex, and Physical Activity Level - 2015-2020 Dietary Guidelines. Accessed June 21, 2020. https://health.gov/our-work/food-nutrition/2015-2020-dietary-guidelines/guidelines/appendix-2/.

"Eating Disorders." National Institute of Mental Health. Accessed June 21, 2020. http://www.nimh.nih.gov/health/topics/eating-disorders/index.shtml.

"FAQs." FAQs | Nutrition.gov. Accessed June 21, 2020. https://www.nutrition.gov/faqs.

"Force-Vector Training." Science for Sport. March 25, 2020. Accessed June 21, 2020. https://www.scienceforsport.com/force-vector-training/.

"Glute Training Program." Around the Clock Fitness. March 14, 2019. Accessed June 21, 2020. http://myaroundtheclockfitness. com/without-moving-a-muscle/.

Jay, Written By:. "Movement Patterns: Horizontal & Vertical Push & Pull Exercises." A Workout Routine. January 20, 2018. Accessed June 21, 2020. https://www.aworkoutroutine. com/movement-patterns/.

Loturco, Irineu, Bret Contreras, Ronaldo Kobal, Victor Fernandes, Neilton Moura, Felipe Siqueira, Ciro Winckler, Timothy Suchomel, and Lucas Adriano Pereira. "Vertically and Horizontally Directed Muscle Power Exercises: Relationships with Top-level Sprint Performance." *Plos One* 13, no. 7 (2018). doi:10.1371/journal.pone.0201475.

Lăcătuşu, Cristina-Mihaela, Elena-Daniela Grigorescu, Mariana Floria, Alina Onofriescu, and Bogdan-Mircea Mihai. "The Mediterranean Diet: From an Environment-Driven Food Culture to an Emerging Medical Prescription." International Journal of Environmental Research and Public Health. March 15, 2019. Accessed June 21, 2020. https://www.ncbi.nlm.nih. gov/pmc/articles/PMC6466433/.

"Mediterranean Diet: MedlinePlus Medical Encyclopedia." MedlinePlus. Accessed April 21, 2020. https://medlineplus. gov/ency/patientinstructions/000110.htm.

"Mediterranean-style Diets Linked to Better Brain Function in Older Adults." ScienceDaily. July 25, 2017. Accessed June 21, 2020. https://www.sciencedaily.com/releases/2017/07/170725154208.htm.

Schoenfeld, B., B. Contreras, D. Ogborn, A. Galpin, J. Krieger, and G. Sonmez. "Effects of Varied Versus Constant Loading Zones on Muscular Adaptations in Trained Men." *International Journal of Sports Medicine*37, no. 06 (2016): 442-47. doi:10.1055/s-0035-1569369.

Schoenfeld, Brad J., and Bret Contreras. "Attentional Focus for Maximizing Muscle Development." *Strength and Conditioning Journal*38, no. 1 (2016): 27-29. doi:10.1519/ssc.0000000000000190.

www.ingramcontent.com/pod-product-compliance
Lightning Source LLC
Chambersburg PA
CBHW062121040426
42336CB00041B/2225